Let Your Mouth Decide

Rah Virgo

BFF
PUBLISHING
HOUSE

Printed in the United States of America

Website: www.rahrahcaters.com

Email: Rahrahcaters@gmail.com

Cover Design: Dominique Stanley

ISBN: 978-1-7352848-0-4

BFF Publishing House is a Limited Liability Corporation dedicated wholly to the appreciation and publication of children and adults for the advancement of diversification in literature.

For more information on publishing contact:

Antionette Mutcherson at
bff@bffpublishinghouse.com
Website: bffpublishinghouse.com
Published in the United States by
BFF Publishing House
Atlanta, Georgia First Edition, 2020

This book is dedicated to my daughter, Ky'mirah Lora, you are the solace in my life. You are the reason I strive to achieve more and build up my legacy. You are the sole reason why I aim to achieve more and more each day. You are GOD's blessing to me. You are the reason I aim to live healthier so that I may live longer. I love you, Kiki!

-Rah Virgo (Mom)

Table of Contents

Vegan Butter

Prep Time: 5 min.

Total Time: 5 min.

Yields: 275 g./9.6 oz.

Ingredients:

1 C. (240 ml.) refined coconut oil, melted (must be refined, not extra virgin)

2 tbsp. avocado oil

1/3 C. (80 ml.) unsweetened soy or almond milk

1 tsp. apple cider vinegar

1 tsp. nutritional yeast

Dash of turmeric

½ tsp. of salt

Process:

1. Add melted refined coconut oil to the blender, along with the avocado oil.
2. Add the apple cider vinegar to the unsweetened almond milk. Make sure to STIR IT IN so that it curdles into a buttermilk-like consistency.
3. Add the yeast, turmeric, and salt.
4. Blend very well until smooth.
5. Pour out into a butter dish and refrigerate until set.
6. Remove from the fridge to thaw for a few minutes. If you want to use it right away on fresh bread or combine it with sugar for baking.

Storage:

Vegan butter lasts for up to two weeks in the fridge. If you want to use it longer, put it in the freezer to store and take out only the desired amount you wish to use.

Coconut Butter

Prep Time: 15 min.

Total Time: 30 min

Yields: 1 & ¼ C.

Creamy coconut butter that's super easy and quick to make!

Ingredients:

4 C. (320 g.) desiccated coconut (shredded, finely grated coconut)

1 tbsp. coconut oil, melted

Process:

1. Add 3 Cups (C.) of the desiccated coconut to the food processor and begin processing. After about 3-4 min., it will start to look a bit sparse, which is when you will add the remaining cup of coconut.

2. Continue to process the coconut. As it starts to form into bits of clumps, add the coconut oil as the machine is still running and keep processing the mixture until it forms a liquid.

3. Turn the Vitamix or blender off and scrape the machine down all sides. Turn the machine back on until the mixture reaches a total liquid consistency. This should take about 15 min. in total.

4. Once the butter has reached liquid consistency in the food processor, it will have a GRAINY texture. This is totally normal and it's fine to use the butter exactly like this.

5. If you want the butter to be mostly or entirely smooth, you can blend it again for another 2 min. to smoothen it to your liking!

Storage:

When finished, store in a sealed mason jar at room temperature. It may harden; if it does, just stand the jar in a bowl or pot of hot water and allow it to melt.

This butter lasts about 2 weeks!

Make sure to date it, VEGANS!

Vegan Parmesan Cheese:

Prep Time: 5 min.

Total Time: 5 min.

Yields: 2 C.

Ingredients:

1 C. cashews

¼ C. nutritional yeast

2 tbsp. hemp seeds

2 tbsp. sesame seeds

2 tbsp. garlic powder

Salt/pepper to taste

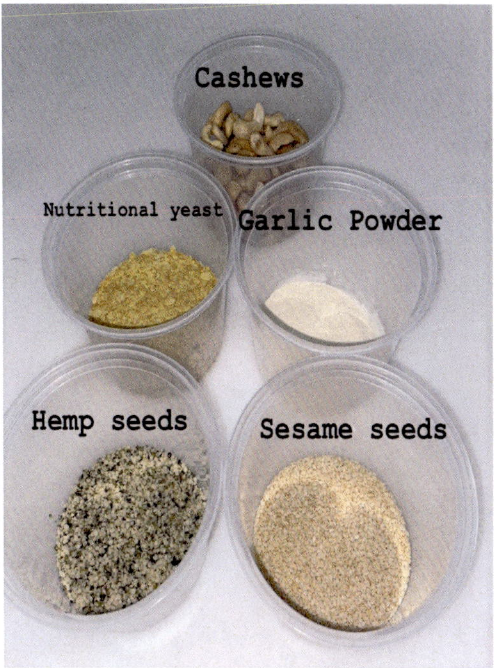
Cashews
Nutritional yeast
Garlic Powder
Hemp seeds
Sesame seeds

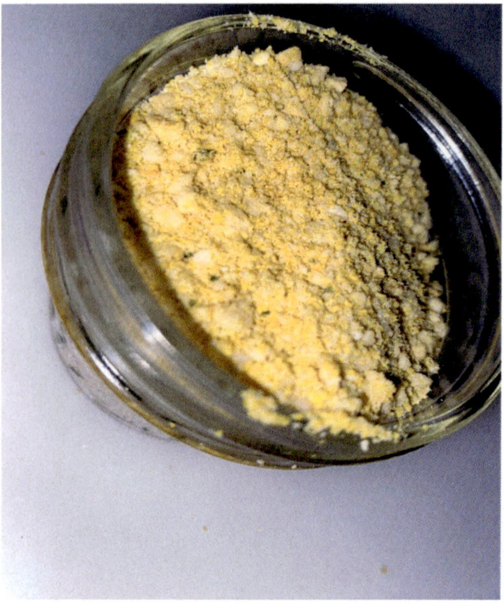

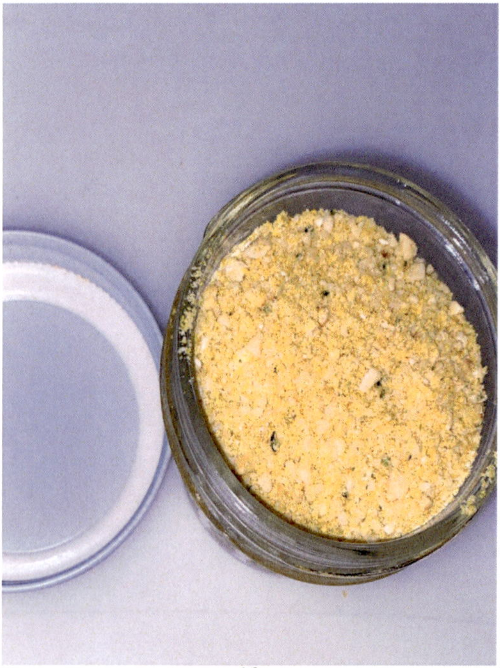

Process:

Add all ingredients to a food processor and run the processor until you have a crumble like consistency.

Storage:

Keep cheese stored in the fridge for up to 30 days in a mason jar or other any glass container you have. Make sure to label and date the jar.

Vegan Buttermilk

Prep Time: 1 hour & 5 min.

Total Time: 1 hour & 5 min.

Yields: 1 Pint

Ingredients:

1 C. raw cashews

1 ¼ C. fresh (filtered) water

2 tbsp. lemon juice or apple cider vinegar

1/8 tsp. Kosher salt (optional)

Process:

1. Place the cashews in a bowl and cover them by at least 1 inch. Let soak for about 1 hour, but the duration yielding the best results is 2 hours.
2. Drain the cashews, and then transfer the nuts to the Vitamix or NutriBullet.
3. Add the water, lemon juice, or apple cider. Add vinegar and salt, then blend the mixture until it is smooth and creamy.

Storage:

Store in a sealed container in the fridge immediately! Lasts between 14-20 days.

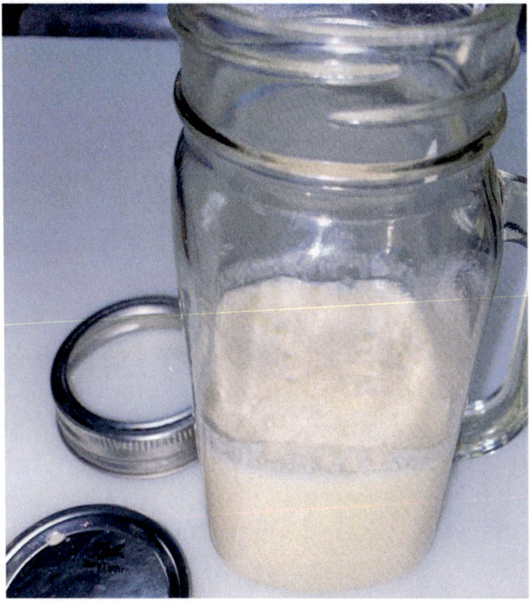

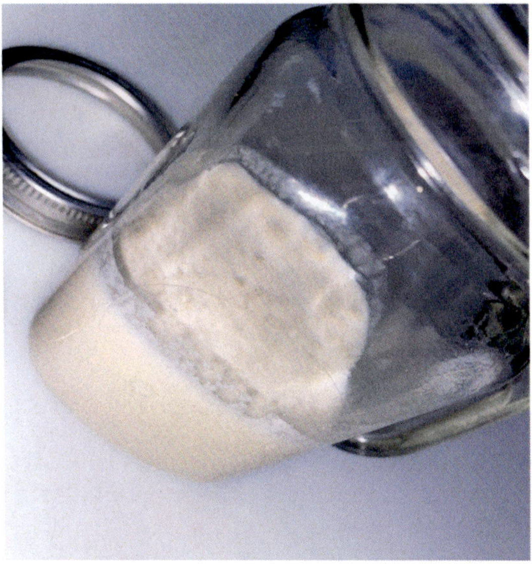

Vegan Mayo

Prep time: 5 min.

Total: 5 min.

Yields: 1 ½ C.

This recipe is very simple, but very easy to mess up! All ingredients, including the non-dairy milk, should be at room temperature! In addition, an immersion blender is the best type of blender for this mix to get it fully emulsified. (This mayonnaise lasts about 5 days. If you will not eat much, please reduce the ingredients by half.

Ingredients:

1 C. (240 ml.) avocado oil

½ C. (120 ml.) unsweetened soy milk ***(can use unsweetened almond milk, but the mayo will not be as creamy!)***

1 tbsp. olive oil

½ tsp. salt

2 tsp. white vinegar

1 tbsp. maple syrup (may use agave as a substitute)

Note: It is crucial that the non-dairy milk is unsweetened. Using sweetened milk will give the mayonnaise a very odd aftertaste.

Process:

Add all of the ingredients to a bowl or measuring jug. Use an immersion blender (handheld) blender to blend it into mayonnaise.

Storage:

Store in a sealed container in the fridge immediately! Lasts between 5 -7 days.

Vegan Buttermilk Fried Mushroom Sandwich

Prep Time: 10 min.

Cook Time: 20 min.

Total Time: 30 min.

Yields: 4 servings

Ingredients:

4 small portobello mushrooms

1 C. non-dairy milk (almond milk, cashew milk, hemp milk)

1 tsp. apple cider Vinegar

¾ C. all-purpose flour

½ C. corn starch

1 tsp. salt

2 tsp. garlic powder

1 tsp. onion powder

¼ tsp. black pepper

Avocado oil for frying (or oil of your choice)

½ C. vegan mayo

1 tbsp. agave syrup

½ tsp. hot sauce

Shredded cabbage

Bun or bread of your choice

Process:

1. Cut the stem out of the portobello mushrooms and make sure they are basically flat. If a mushroom has a large curve on its edge, please be sure to trim it so that it's flat.

2. Whisk together your almond milk and apple cider vinegar. It should sit until it begins to curdle, which is now the buttermilk (as per recipe seen on page 14).

3. In a medium-sized mixing bowl, combine corn starch, flour, salt, pepper, garlic, and onion powder. Then, combine the buttermilk into the dry mixture and whisk until it is fully incorporated with no lumps.

4. Heat the oil on medium-high heat in a large cast-iron skillet (or any pan of your choice). There should be about ½ an inch of oil in the pan. Once the pan is hot, dip a mushroom into your batter and begin the coating process. The mushroom should be coated completely.

5. Gently—not too hard, you don't want any hot oil popping onto your skin—place the mushroom in oil fry on one side until it is nice and golden brown, about 2-3 min. You will then flip the mushroom and fry it on the other side for a few moments until the whole thing is brown and crispy.

6. Repeat step 5 with all of the mushrooms. Once they are done, place them on a paper towel and sprinkle them with a dash more of salt.

7. Make the mayonnaise by whisking together the vegan mayonnaise, agave, and hot sauce.

8. Finally, put together your tasty sandwiches: a little bit of mayonnaise on the bun, then mushroom cabbage or any type of green you would like, and more mayonnaise if you choose. Serve immediately!

Vegan Scalloped Potatoes

Prep Time: 30 min.

Cook time: 1 hour

Total Time: 1 hour and 30 min.

Yields: 4-6 Servings

Ingredients:

4 lbs. Yukon gold potatoes

1 tbsp. olive oil

1 large onion, sliced thin

4 large garlic cloves, minced

Vegan Parmesan (***feel free to refer to page 2 for Parmesan recipe***) for garnish, chopped chives

Cream Sauce:

1 ½ C. raw cashews, soaked in hot water 5 min. prior

2 C. veg. broth

2 C. coconut milk or unsweetened non-dairy milk

½ C. nutritional yeast

2 tsp. salt

1 tsp. onion powder

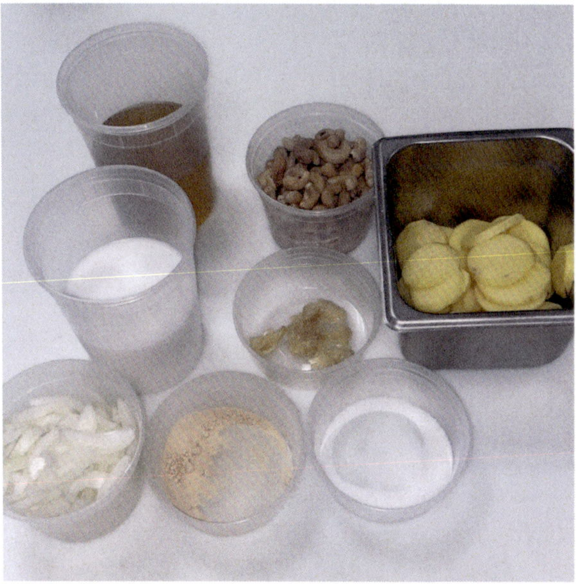

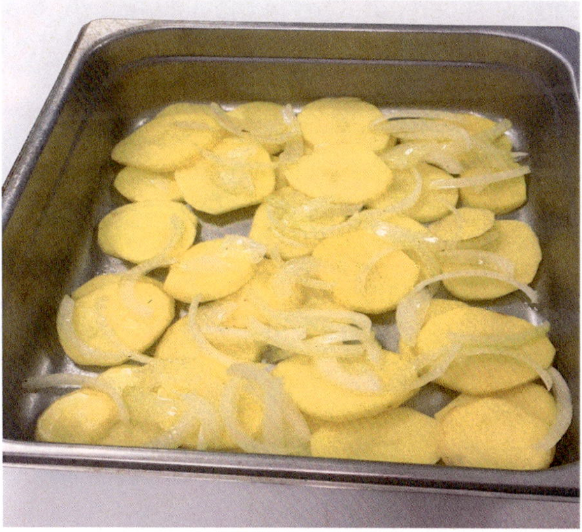

Process:

1. Peel your potatoes, slice into 1/8 inch thick rounds. Try to cut all of the potatoes to the same desired thickness so that all potatoes cook evenly. Preheat the oven to 375 degrees Fahrenheit and lightly grease a 9 x 13 inchbaking dish, or you can lightly spray with Pam. Set aside.

2. For the sauce: In a high-powered blender, such as a Vitamix or Ninja blender, add all of the sauce ingredients and blend on high for about 4 min. or until smooth.

3. Heat the olive oil in a large sauté pan over medium heat. Add the sliced onion and sauté for about 3-4 min., ONLY until translucent. Then, add the garlic to the pan and let cook for only 1 min., stirring constantly. Turn off heat and set aside.

4. Spread ½ of sliced potatoes in the baking dish. Top evenly with half of the cream sauce, then add the onion/garlic mix on top of the cream sauce.

5. Layer the rest of the potatoes and the rest of the sauce. Put in the oven for about 60 min. until it is fork-tender, If it is not tender, stick it back in the oven for another 10-20 min. The sauce should be bubbly and thick.

6. Once done, let sit for about 30 min. to cook and condense all flavors. Slice and enjoy!

Storage: Lasts for about 5 days.

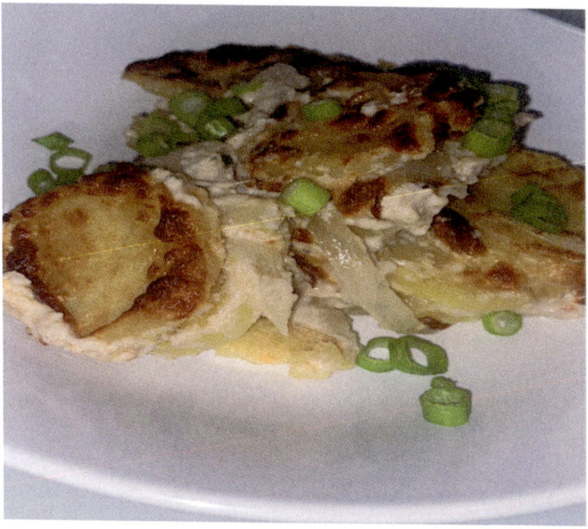

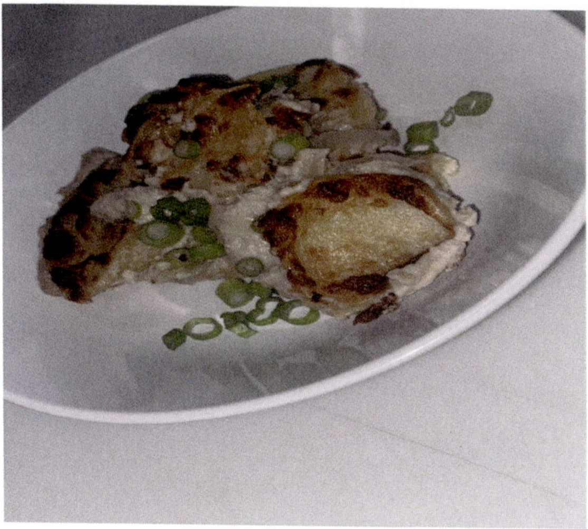

Chickpea Stew

Prep Time: 22 min.

Cook Time: 40 min.

Total Time:1 hr & 2 min.

Yields: 6 servings

Ingredients:

½ tsp. basil, dried

1 carrot

2 garlic cloves

1 onion medium

½ tsp. oregano, dried

1 tbsp. parsley, dried

¼ C. red bell pepper

1 tomato

2 C. veggie broth

4 tbsp. tomato paste

¼ tsp. cayenne pepper

½ tsp. chili flakes

2 tbsp. of your favorite hot sauce

½ tsp. salt

1 tbsp. olive oil

1 C. dry chickpeas or two 15 oz. cans (note: make sure to drain the liquid).

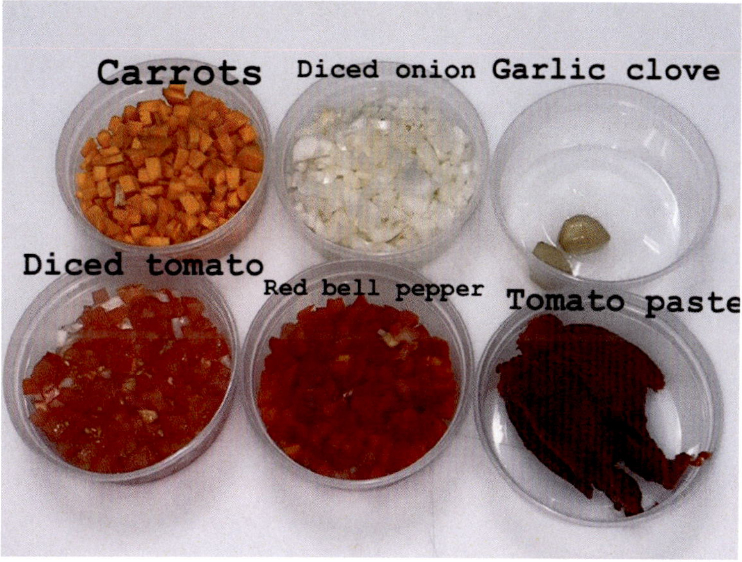

Process:

1. Try to use chickpeas in a can. If using dried chickpeas, soak overnight, then drain and rinse the next day.
2. Cover chickpeas with water about 2 inches above the chickpeas. Bring to a boil on medium heat.
3. Lower heat to a simmer and cook until tender for about 45 min. to an hour.
4. Drain the chickpeas of water and set aside. **If using canned chickpeas, start at this step:**
5. Heat oil or water in a large saucepan on medium-high heat. Add onion and cook until translucent, about 4 min.
6. Add garlic and cook for about 40 seconds, constantly stirring. Add bell pepper, tomatoes, carrots, chickpeas, parsley, basil, and oregano.
7. Add tomato paste and vegetable broth, cover, and bring to a boil. Reduce to a simmer for 20-30 min. or until thickened.
8. Mash some of the chickpeas with the back of a fork to thicken the stew.
9. Check the seasoning. Add your cayenne pepper and hot sauce, as well as a dash of salt and pepper to taste as needed.
10. Serve with brown rice and enjoy!

Storage: Freeze for desired lentgh of time.

Recipe Notes: This here is one of my best sellers! I hope that you enjoy all the flavors!

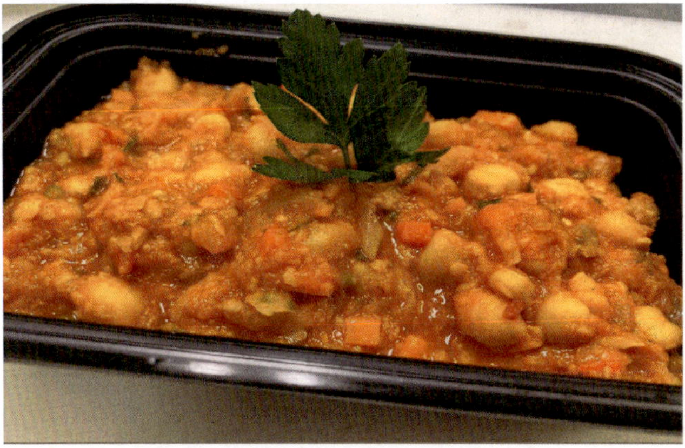

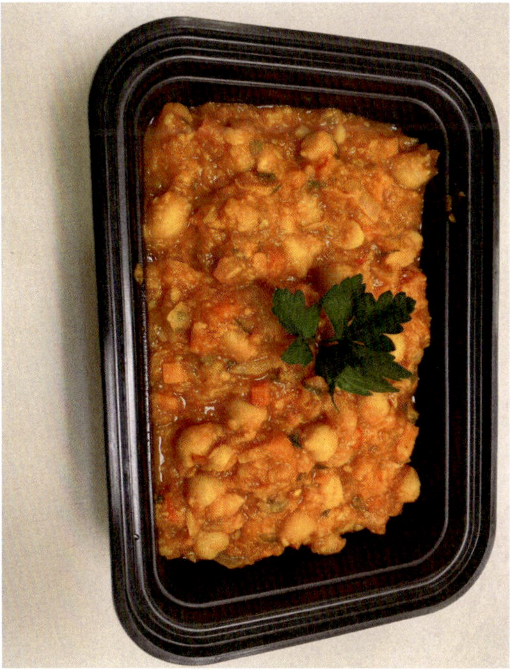

Sweet Potato, Chickpea, & Spinach Coconut Curry

Prep Time: 25 min.

Cook Time: 25 min.

Total Time: 50 min.

Yields: 10 Servings

Ingredients:

One 15 oz. can of chickpeas

1 tomato, diced small

One 5 oz. package of baby spinach

1 bunch of cilantro (fresh leaves)

1 tsp. coriander, ground

3 garlic cloves

4 tsp. fresh ginger

1 lime

1 onion, diced small (should measure into about 2 C.)

1 sweet potato (medium or large)

1 can of light coconut milk (14 oz.)

1 C. of basmati rice, cooked

1 tsp. black pepper cracked

¼ tsp. red pepper flakes

¾ sea salt, fine

1 tsp. turmeric, ground

4 tsp. virgin coconut oil

1 tbsp. cumin seeds or ground cumin

3 tbsp. curry powder

1 tbsp. coconut flakes, unsweetened

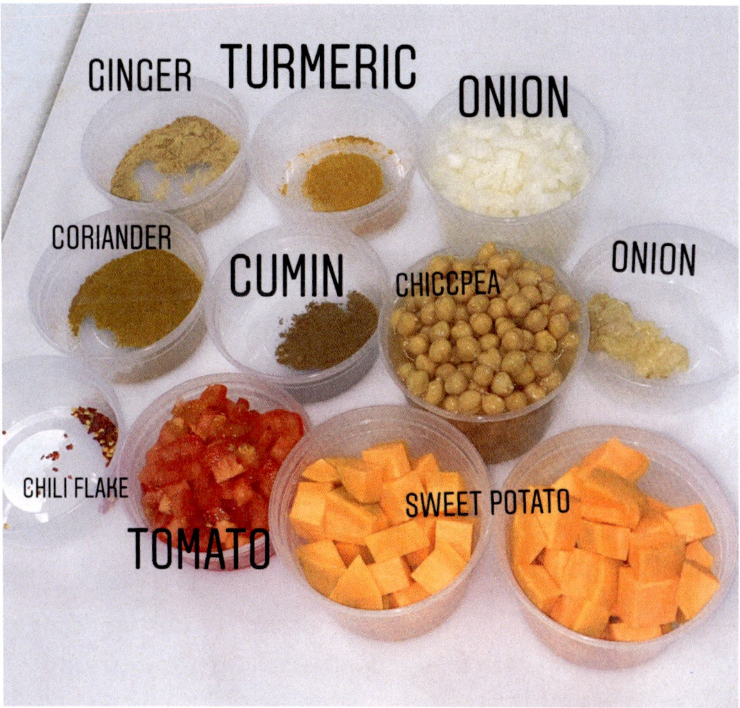

Process:

1. In a large saucepan, heat the oil over medium heat. Add one cumin seed in the pan and make sure it sizzles. Once it does, the pan is HOT! Add the cumin seeds and toast for about 1 min., until there is a lightly fragrant smell and the seeds are dark in color. Be careful not to burn them. Toast the seeds for literally only 1 min. Immediately afterwards, stir in the onion and season with a pinch of salt. Cook for about 4-5 min. until the onion is soft and translucent.

2. Add the garlic, ginger, turmeric, curry, coriander, and red pepper flakes. Sauté until the garlic softens a bit.

3. I suggest cooking the sweet potato separately for about 15 min., so it's properly cooked before going to the next step!

4. Add the sweet potato, chickpeas, tomatoes with the juices as well from when you cut this helps a lot for flavor and coconut milk. Stir to combine, cover and simmer over medium heat for about 20-30 min., until the potatoes are fork tender.

5. **Optional step:** get a potato masher and mash ⅓ of the mix just to thicken up the sauce.

6. Stir in the spinach and cook until wilted. Season with salt and pepper to taste.

7. Serve on a bed of cooked grains, such as quinoa or rice. Garnish with fresh chopped cilantro and coconut flakes. Squeeze lime over the entire dish to extract all of the flavors. YUM!

Storage: Freeze for desired lentgh of time omitting rice.

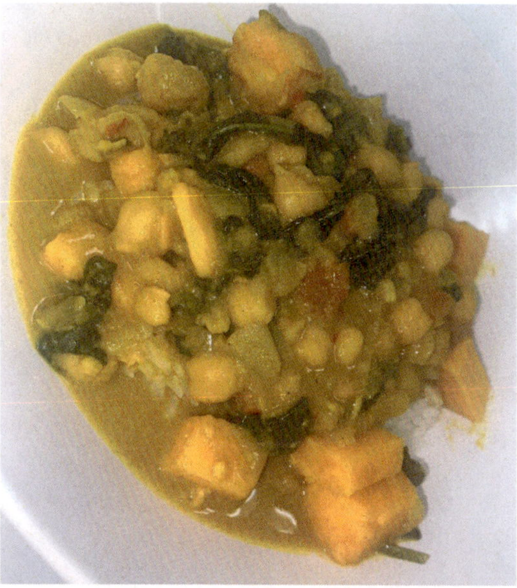

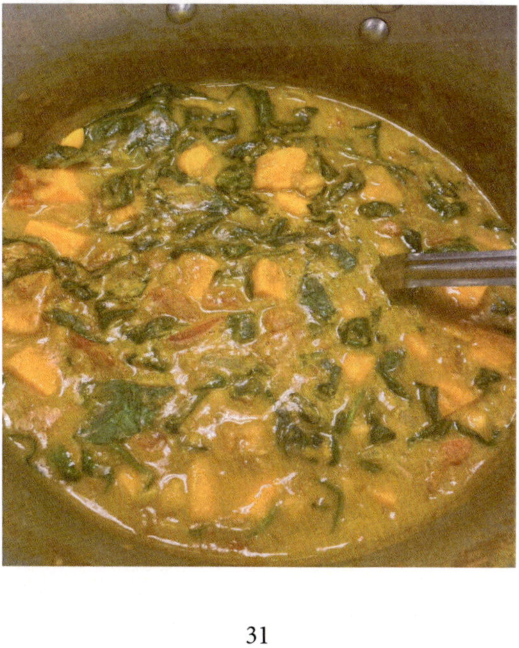

Mushroom Risotto

Prep Time: 15 min.

Cook Time: 40 min.

Total Time: 55 min.

Ingredients: 10

Yields: 2 servings (double batch if you want 4 servings)

Ingredients:

100 g. white button mushrooms or Shiitake, whichever you prefer (sliced thin)

3 garlic cloves

1 fresh parsley

4-6 sprigs of fresh thyme

1 small shallot, diced

500 ml. veg stock

1 ½ C. white wine

100 g. arborio rice

4 tbsp. nutritional yeast flakes

1 tbsp. salt & pepper (adjust to taste)

1 tbsp. olive oil

½ tbsp. white wine vinegar (optional)

Notes: dairy-free, gluten-free, nut-free, soy-free

Process:

1. Remove thyme from sprigs, set aside.
2. Dice shallot very finely, set aside.
3. Dice garlic cloves very finely, set aside.
4. Chop up parsley, set aside.
5. Heat the olive oil in a large sauté pan, add the diced shallot, thyme, and diced garlic clove, cook on low-medium heat until softened.
6. Add in the mushroom and cook until sauté to your liking, generally for about 1-2 min.
7. Stir in the rice, then immediately add white wine to it. Constantly stir with a rubber spatula. Cover and let cook for about 5 min., turning the heat down.
8. Immediately return to the pan and add veg. stock—this is where it gets tricky. Add veg stock ladle by ladle. Each time you do this, make sure that the stock is completely cooked and dissolved in rice. Once dissolved, add another ladle and keep doing so until there is no more veg stock. Cover your rice each time on low-medium heat. Let cook for about 15-20 min. The rice should be very soft, melting-in-your-mouth soft. When finished, top with fresh parsley and serve!

Storage: Last up to four days in thr fridge.

Notes:

You can adjust with more vegtable stock if the rice isn't fully cooked and use lower heat. Please keep covered at all times! Very important!

Towards the last seven minutes of cooking, add in nutritional yeast for a cheesy flavor. This is optional, for the dish works without it as well.

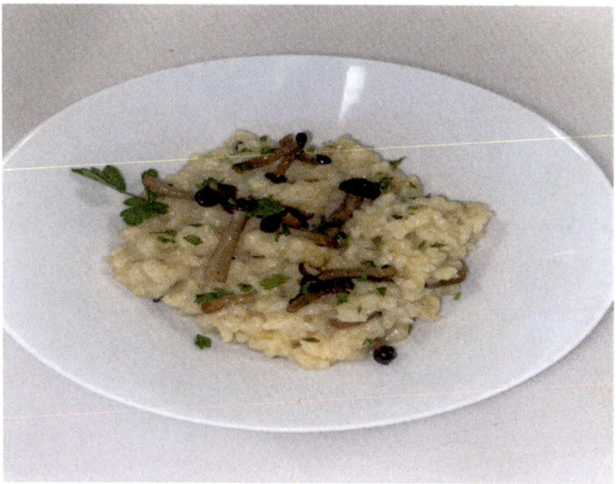

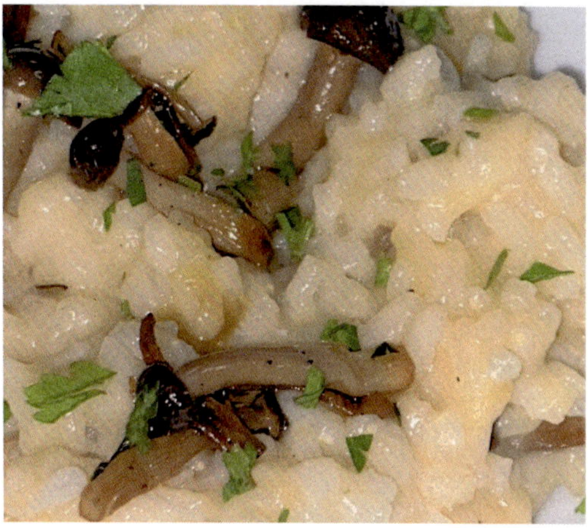

Vegan Corn Chowder

Prep Time: 15 min.

Cook Time: 40 min.

Total Time: 55 min.

Yields: 4 Servings

Ingredients:14

3 carrots, large

2 large red potatoes peeled and chopped

3 large stalks celery diced

4 ears corn shucked and steamed

5 large garlic cloves minced

1 red bell pepper large cored and chopped

1 white onion, large

2/3 c. coconut milk

2 tsp. Cajun seasoning

½ tsp. paprika

1 ½ tsp. sea salt

3 tbsp. coconut oil

¼ tsp. cumin, ground

2 c. water

This recipe contains no heavy cream or butter but it tastes so rich and decadent, YUM! It's sort of like a chowder with benefits. Try to get fresh corn as possible while in season.

Process:

1. Place ears of corn into large pot and fill with water drop about 2 tablespoons of salt. Cover pot with lid and place over high heat on stove. Bring to a boil and cook until corn is plump and juicy about a good 5-8 minutes.

2. Remove corn from pot, it's a good idea to use tongs while doing so and place on cutting board.

3. Chop one of the red potatoes in half and place it in the same pot of boiling water you used to cook the corn. Allow potato to cook until fork tender about 10-15 minutes.

4. While potato is cooking, sauté the rest of your vegetables. In a large pot add coconut oil, along with the other diced potato, chopped onion, garlic, carrots, celery, bell pepper, sea salt, Cajun seasoning, paprika and cumin. Turn the heat to medium-high and sauté, stirring occasionally until vegetables have softened about 10-12 minutes.

5. Use a knife to remove the corn kernels from all of the ears of corn. Place half of the kernels in a blender, along with the cooked potato. Add the coconut milk and water (or your broth) to the blender and blend until completely smooth. You may have to blend a good 2-3 times until completely smooth.

6. Add the remaining corn kernels to the pot with the sautéed vegetables, and then pour the blended corn/ potato chowder mixture into the pot. Bring to a gentle boil and cook until potato has been softened fully, which will be about 10-20 minutes.
7. Remove from heat and taste chowder. Add sea salt and Cajun seasoning and adjust to your taste. Serve with chopped green onion. Enjoy.

Storage: Lasts 3-5 days in the fridge.

Honey Garlic Cauliflower

Prep time: 16 min.

Cook Time: 27 min.

Total Time: 43 min.

Serving: 4

Ingredients:

1 small head of cauliflower (in which you will cut into bite size florets)

3 c. panko bread crumbs

Cooking oil spray (Pam works just fine)

2 large eggs whisked

1-2 scallions, finely sliced

Sauce:

6 tbsp. honey

5 garlic cloves minced

1 tsp. onion powder

6 tbsp. water + 2tsp cornstarch

2 tbsp. low sodium soy sauce

2 tbsp. siracha sauce

Process:

1. Preheat the oven to 350 F. Line a baking sheet or tray with parchment paper. Spread across the bread crumbs evenly across the surface of the baking sheet. You then heavily spray the bread crumbs with the cooking oil spray. Bake crumbs about 5-7 minutes, or until golden brown. SHOULD NOT bake more than 10 minutes!

2. Whisk the eggs, set aside in a small bowl. Line another baking tray or sheet with parchment paper.

3. After cutting cauliflower into florets, you're going to dip cauliflower in egg mixture then shake it multiple times to make sure the excess egg drip off. This part is key due to the fact you do not want your breadcrumbs overly wet from too much egg mix. Nor will the bread crumbs stick to the cauliflower. Next cover the egg battered cauliflower with bread crumbs.

4. Place coated cauliflower on an empty tray with no parchment and stick in oven for about 25 minutes or until cauliflower is fully cooked and the coating is dark golden brown. You can also check the stem of the floret if it is soft it is time to pull from the oven! No one likes a super hard cauliflower!

5. While cauliflower is baking, make sauce on stove top. Start with a small ball by completely dissolving the cornstarch and water mix, then setting aside.

6. Add all sauce ingredients except the cornstarch slurry mix to a small pot or sauce pan. Bring up to a soft gentle simmer all while stirring or whisking until all ingredients are thoroughly mixed. Sauce should become a dark golden brown. You're then going to add your cornstarch slurry. While pouring in whisk to get it fully incorporated.

7. Next your going to let the sauce come up to a simmer after pouring in slurry the sauce should be a golden brown boiling up. Once this happens the sauce is done you can fully drizzle sauce over cauliflower. If want a heavy coating I say grab a pastry brush and put on top of cauliflower.
8. Lastly, The scallions you chopped up garnish the cauliflower with them.

Notes: This is my second-best seller! Enjoy this simple but cultural dish!

Lentil Pasta With Vegan Butter & Garlic Sauce

Prep Time: 5 min.

Cook Time-10-12 min.

Total: 15- 17 min.

Yield: 6 servings

Ingredients:

12 oz. bag Red Lentil Pasta

8 cloves of garlic (minced)

4 tbsp Vegan Butter (use recipe from page 1 or earth balance at local supermarket)

1 tbsp. garlic powder

1 tbsp. onion powder

1 tsp. Cajun seasoning

Salt/pepper to taste

10 oz. broccoli steamed or boiled your choice

Vegan Parmesan cheese to top (use recipe from page 10)

Process:

1. Cook minced garlic, oil, butter and all spices including salt and pepper in a skillet over medium heat for about 5 minutes, or just as the garlic browns a bit.

2. Prepare lentil pasta according to your package instructions. While your pasta and sauce is being prepped make your steamed broccoli. This process should take about 10-12 minutes for your florets to become tender.

3. Once everything is done pour into one bowl and mix until well incorporated. Season with more salt, pepper, Cajun if desired and top with the Vegan Parm. and enjoy!

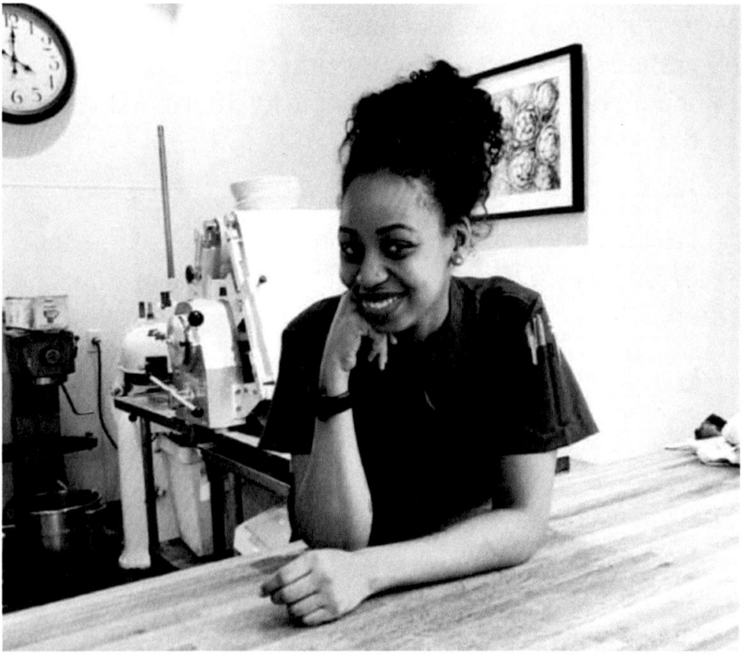

Rah Virgo

WWW.RAHRAHCATERS.COM
RAHRAHCATERS@GMAIL.COM

Made in United States
Orlando, FL
04 November 2026

90201276R00029